Lavender Essential Oil

LISA BARGER

Cover Design: Amy Jambor

Photo Credit: BigStockPhoto.com/VitalinaRybakova

ISBN: 1517416183
ISBN-13: 978-1517416188

WHO I AM & WHY I WROTE THIS BOOK

It's easily the most popular of all the volatile organic compounds we know as essential oils. And it's no wonder. After all, lavender is widely available, relatively inexpensive and listed among the safest of all volatile oils. Lavender essential oil is truly beloved by aroma professionals and enthusiasts alike.

Esoteric practitioners teach that the scent of lavender deepens meditation, enhances concentration and brings the body's energies into balance. They use lavender essential oil to improve their patients' moods, reduce anxiety and lower blood pressure.

Professional aromatherapists believe that distilled lavender is analgesic, anti-inflammatory and antispasmodic. They know that it kills harmful bacteria, viruses and fungi and use it to treat skin conditions like eczema and dandruff.

But this book wasn't written for them. This book was created for you.

My name is Lisa Barger. I am a master herbalist who has spent the past twenty years sharing what I know about herbs and herbal remedies, essential oils, and "alternative" therapies like Bach flower remedies, Tai Chi, acupuncture and more.

I am the founder of, and principle writer for, a network of websites covering everything from herbal remedies to pet food recalls. I cover the good and the bad of "natural" health--and expose the bogus.

But I'm also the author of several books. My books on essential oils include titles like *Dangerous Aromatherapy*, *How Essential Oils Are Made* and *Aromatherapy Lists*.

I wrote those books because, to be blunt, I had exhausted the aromatherapy books written by today's most recognizable aroma authors and wanted more. Dismissive comments like "They say," and "Studies show," weren't enough for me. I wanted to know who "they" were; I wanted to read the studies for myself. But somehow, most of our popular aromatherapy authors never quite get around to including that information.

I felt cheated and I wondered what the big secret was.

And that is why I wrote those books.

In *Lavender Essential Oil*, you'll read about the four species of lavender that make up nearly all the lavender essential oil on the market today:

- *Lavandula angustifolia*
- *Lavandula dentata*
- *Lavandula latifolia*
- *Lavandula stoechas*

I'll share with you the history of lavender, show you how modern herbalists use both the herb and its volatile oils and then give you real-life examples of the scientific study being done on lavender.

And because the people who use lavender oil are as diverse as the species from which it is distilled, you'll learn how lavender is used in the three major branches of aromatherapy:

- Medical aromatherapy
- Emotional aromatherapy
- Holistic aromatherapy

But you'll go even deeper. You'll debunk the myth that "doctors don't use herbs" when you see that lavender is, in fact, being studied. You'll walk away with the scientific citations so that, if you choose to, you can look up the actual studies for yourself. No vague "they say" and "studies prove" nonsense here. You'll see exactly who "they" are and exactly what they "say".

Lavender Essential Oil was written to give you information you might not find in other aromatherapy books. It isn't a medical text—and it shouldn't be used as one—but it does take an in-depth look at what is arguably the most important product in the healing art we call aromatherapy.

I know there are a lot of quicky, junk books out there and the field of aromatherapy certainly offers its share of them. *Lavender Essential Oil* is different. I thank you for reading it.

~ Lisa Barger

"Tiny, dried petals rustled out of the meshes, for Miss Ainslie's laces were laid away in lavender, like her love." ~ *Lavender and Old Lace*, Myrtle Reed

CONTENTS

THIS BOOKLET IS NOT A MEDICAL TEXT

Lavender Essential Oil is not a medical text; nothing in this booklet is intended as medical advice. It is not the author's intention to encourage self-diagnosis or self-treatment of any medical condition.

Lavender Essential Oil references scientific studies on the volatile organic compounds we refer to as "essential oils". A scientific study—even a positive one—is not proof that lavender essential oil is safe or effective for any particular medical issue.

ABOUT THIS BOOKLET'S BINOMIALS

Botany is an evolving science; plants are renamed and even moved into different (or new) genera as better information becomes available. Whenever the author had to choose among multiple botanical names, she chose the binomial currently accepted by the world's botanical authorities. This book's botanical names may differ from those in texts you already own.

ABOUT THIS BOOKLET'S REFERENCES

This booklet was written for the aromatherapy enthusiast who cannot be satisfied with "they say" and "studies show". In that spirit, the author has chosen a streamlined format for *Lavender Essential Oil*'s references.

FINANCIAL DISCLOSURE

Neither Lisa Barger nor anyone associated with the LisaBarger.com family of websites or Lisa Barger Publishing has any financial relationship to any person or business referenced in this booklet.

In 2003 Ms. Barger was a one-time wholesale client of Amrita Aromatherapy.

OUR LOVE AFFAIR WITH LAVENDER

Why is the entire aromatherapy world so in love with lavender? From a scientific point of view, it's hardly the most important of the volatile organic extracts we call essential oils. It isn't the strongest germ-killer or the most potent antioxidant or the best anti-inflammatory.

And in the garden, lavender isn't even a particularly attractive plant, especially after its blue-purple flowers fade for the season. Its silvery leaves tend to look tired and faded next to the more vibrant greens of mints, thymes and basils. Also, as any home gardener who has grown lavender can tell you, it has an annoying tendency to fall open, leaving the bark at the heart of the plant bare and exposed.

So why are there thousands of blog posts, magazine articles and social media infographics declaring lavender "the only essential oil you'll ever need" and enshrining it at the head of lists of the herbal remedies every home should stock? I believe that lavender's rein as ruler of the aromatherapy world has its feet planted in many gardens.

First, it's a plant with a rich, and colorful, history. Lavender was among the herbs used to prepare Solomon's Temple. Centuries later it fought plague in Europe. And it was lavender that the father of aromatherapy, René-Maurice Gatafossé, successfully used to treat his burned hand after it became gangrenous. Nicholas Culpepper said of lavender it was, "so well known it needs no description." Maud Grieve, in her guidebook, *A Modern Herbal,* devoted seven pages to it.

Lavender oil is equally beloved. No other essential oil can match lavender in its sheer versatility. Today's aromatherapy authors recommend lavender essential oil for just about everything from soothing colic to wound care to easing post-chemotherapy sickness.

It is a favorite scent in both personal care and cleaning products; you'll find lavender used to scent soap, shampoo, body wash, lotion, diaper rash ointment, laundry soaps, dishwashing liquids, carpet powders . . . if it is stocked in your pharmacy's toiletry or cleaning aisles, it probably comes in a lavender scent.

Lavender hydrosols, which are natural byproducts of the essential oil distillation process, are packaged for sale as facial toners, body sprays and fabric fresheners.

Science loves lavender, too. In 2015 alone lavender was studied as a sleep aid, an anxiety reducer and a heart protector. And though it isn't allergen-free, as some essential oil distributors claim, lavender consistently ranks among the volatile extracts considered safest for most people.

Also contributing to lavender's popularity is its unique ability to smell just medicinal enough. It is as if lavender evolved just to beckon users with a simple promise: "I'm powerful but I'm still livable."

So how do you fully exploit the gifts that lavender offers? Understanding why all lavender oils are not created (or distilled) equally is the key to choosing the particular essential oil that is best for you.

THE FOUR LAVENDERS OF AROMATHERAPY

The genus *Lavandula* offers us thirty-nine officially recognized species of lavender but only four, *Lavandula angustifolia*, *Lavandula latifolia*, *Lavandula dentata* and *Lavandula stoechas* are routinely found in modern aromatherapy.

Although all four are native to the Mediterranean each species was known to the healers of old; each has its own centuries-old history of use in folk medicine.

But perhaps it is the essential oil that is most prized these days. Lavender oil, regardless of its exact botanical source, is always distilled from the flowers and leaves of the parent plant. The very best oil, say aromatherapists, comes from plants grown at the highest altitudes possible in France. Aficionados go even further and demand that only the flowers be distilled—and that the water is never allowed to actually reach a true boil.

LAVANDULA ANGUSTIFOLIA

Botanical Name: *Lavandula angustifolia*
Common Names: English lavender, true lavender, pure lavender
Production Method: Distillation
Materials Used: Flowers, Leaves

Lavandula angustifolia is, for most people, the "real" lavender. This is the species Nicholas Culpepper said was so well-known to the herbalists of his era that it "needs no description"; it is the "lavender vera" of Maud Grieve's famous herbal text and the one most lavender essential oil is made of.

LAVANDULA DENTATA

Botanical Name: *Lavandula dentata*
Common Names: French lavender, fringed lavender
Production Method: Distillation
Materials Used: Flowers, Leaves

The "dentata" part of this lavender's botanical name comes from the Italian word for "toothed". Take one look at the plant's silvery-gray leaves and you'll immediately know why. Also known as French lavender, this species is heavily used in the perfume industry.

LAVANDULA LATIFOLIA

Botanical Name: *Lavandula latifolia*
Common Names: Spike lavender, Portuguese lavender
Production Method: Distillation
Materials Used: Flowers, Leaves

It may not be as well-known as "true" lavender but this species offers a scent that is stronger and a bit more camphorus. Also known as broadleaf lavender—a feature that is referenced in the "*latifolia*" part of its botanical name—Portugese lavender is native to an area running from Portugal to Italy.

LAVANDULA STOECHAS

Botanical Name: *Lavandula stoechas*
Common Names: Spike lavender, Spanish lavender
Production Method: Distillation
Materials Used: Flowers, Leaves

Of the four major lavenders in common usage in aromatherapy, spike lavender is considered to have the harshest aroma. It is rarely chosen just for its scent. However the compounds that "harden" spike's scent also make it more desirable for certain therapeutic treatments.

LAVENDER IN TRADITIONAL HEALING

The various lavenders have a long, long history of use in herbal medicine.

In Ayurveda

In the traditional folk medicine of India, Ayurveda, lavender is categorized as a pungent, sweet and bitter herb. It is used to cool the body and is prized for its ability to reduce both Pitta and Kapha. Digestive, it is considered a pungent remedy and is assigned these values:

- Antispasmodic
- Carminative
- Diuretic

The species most often cited in Ayurvedic herbal texts appears to be *L. angustifolia*, or "true" lavender.

In Traditional Chinese Medicine

No species of *Lavandula* is known to be native to China. Furthermore, essential oils are not typically used in traditional Chinese medicine.

In Bach Flower Therapy

Despite the widespread planting of lavender in the UK, Edward Bach used no species of lavender to produce any of his Bach flower remedies.

In Native American Healing

No species of lavender is native to the Americas so no Native American people is known to have used any lavender product for traditional healing.

In Homeopathy

No species of lavender is used to make succussed homeopathic remedies. Nor is it generally recommended to use essential oils, which are concentrated, alongside homeopathic remedies because the essential oils will overpower the homeopathic medicines, which are, by contrast, very dilute.

In European Herbal Medicine

It is in the herbal medicine systems of Western Europe, where most species of lavender grow naturally, that the herb saw the widest medicinal use. Herbalist John Gerard compared English lavender to other species concluding that it had "a more grateful smell" and recommending it for ailments of the head, especially, because of its "hot and dry" characteristics. In his text The *Herball*, he prescribed distillations of lavender for:

- Cold diseases of the head
- Catalepsy
- Migraine
- Epilepsy
- Fainting
- Panting and passions of the heart
- Giddiness
- Palsy

Fifty years later, another famous herbalist, Nicholas Culpepper, described English lavender as a plant "so well known that it needs no introduction." He then placed it under the sign of Mercury and prescribed it for:

- Apoplexy (especially in the brain)
- Epilepsy
- Edema
- Fainting
- Hoarseness
- Toothache
- Arrhythmia

Culpepper also taught that lavender could bring about menstruation. He prescribed it after a miscarriage to completely empty the uterus.

Of the essential oil, which Culpepper called oil of spike, he wrote it is "so fierce and piercing a quality that it is cautiously to be used". He recommended it for "inward or outward griefs."

Maud Grieve's 1931 *A Modern Herbal* devoted several pages to the various lavenders and the essential oils produced from them. She assigned lavender these properties:

- Aromatic
- Carminative
- Nervine

By the time Grieve wrote her herbal text lavender had largely fallen out of favor as a medicinal herb but it was still used sometimes to cover the scent of ointments and other remedies.

Of the essential oil, Grieve said it was "restorative" and "tonic". A dose of up to 4 drops, she explained, could be added to a bit of sugar or a glass of milk to treat:

- Lack of appetite
- Fallen spirits
- Flatulence

Grieve documented many topical uses for lavender essential oil. As a foot soak, it "has a marked influence in relieving fatigue" and could be applied directly for:

- Toothache
- Neuralgia
- Sprains
- Arthritis

Grieve, like many other herbalists, treated lavender as a stimulant and used it to treat "hysteria", palsy and similar "disorders of debility".

One of Grieve's more unusual uses for lavender is as a way to calm captive lions and tigers. Big cats, she says, "become docile under its influence".

Further Reading About Lavender In Traditional Healing:

Tirtha, S. (1998). *The Ayurveda Encyclopedia.* Ayurveda Holistic Center Press.

Bach, E. (1936). *The Twelve Healers And Other Remedies.* The C. W. Daniel Company Limited. Available online:
http://www.bachcentre.com/centre/download/healers.htm

Gerard, J. (1957). *The Herball, Or Generall Historie Of Plantes.* Available online:
http://www.botanicus.org/title/b12080317

Culpepper, N. (1653). *Complete Herbal.* Available online:
http://www.bibliomania.com/2/1/66/113/frameset.html

Grieve, M. (1931). *A Modern Herbal.* Jonathan Cape.

LAVENDER IN MODERN HERBAL MEDICINE

Lavender may not see the extensive medical use that it once did but it is still employed by today's herbalists. Health agencies like the World Health Organization, The US National Institutes of Health and the European Medicines Agency have all looked at how traditional healers use lavender; many of those agencies have gone on to issue official recommendations about dosage, guidelines on purity and, of course, safety information.

Lavender's Commission E Monograph

Germany's Commission E monograph on lavender defines the flowers and the essential oil distilled from those flowers (but not the leaves) as the therapeutic parts of the parent plant. In respect to dried lavender flowers, the Commission approved them for these ailments:

- Mood disorders
- Insomnia
- Stomach and digestive conditions
- Roemheld syndrome

No side effects, contraindications or drug interactions were noted, although the Commission did say lavender may work best when it is combined with herbs that also have sedative or digestive actions.

A typical dose would be 1 or 2 teaspoons of the dried flowers steeped in a cup of water or up to 100 grams of the flowers added to a bath. For the essential oil, which should be distilled from *L. angustifolia*, up to 4 drops may be placed on a sugar cube.

Lavender's WHO Monograph

The World Health Organization, or WHO, also recognizes lavender oil for several purposes. Traditionally, say the WHO's researchers, lavender oil was used for:

- Burns and wounds
- Diarrhea
- Headache
- Sore throat

The monograph also lists a number of possible therapeutic actions found during various tests on lavender, including, in some tests, the essential oil.

Those potential actions include:

- Antibacterial
- Antioxidant
- Antiulcer
- Sedative
- Uterine stimulant

The accepted dosage is 1 to 2 teaspoons of dried herb made into a tea, which is then taken up to 3 times per day. Externally, up to 100 grams of dried lavender flowers can be used in a bath.

For the essential oil, there is no dosage listed; instead the WHO recognizes a 1:5 tincture taken up to 3 times per day.

Lavender's European Medicines Agency Monograph

The European Medicines Agency formally recognizes lavender essential oil distilled from *L. angustifolia* as both a topical and an oral remedy. It lists no "Well-Established" uses but acknowledges lavender's traditional role in treating conditions like:

- Mental Stress
- Exhaustion
- Sleep disorders

The official dosage is from 20 to 80 milligrams, taken orally or 1 to 3 grams added to a bath lasting up to 20 minutes. Due to lavender oil's believed sedative effects, it should not be used by people who plan to drive or operate machinery.

The oils should not be used, adds the agency, in baths by people who have open or large wounds or acute skin diseases. Nor should it be used by people with high fevers, infections, circulatory problems or heart failure.

Like most essential oils, lavender has not been extensively studied for use in babies and children. The agency notes that lavender essential oil should not be used on children; nor should it be used by lactating mothers.

Lavender & The US National Institutes Of Health

The National Institutes of Health recognizes lavender essential oil as "possibly effective" for only a few uses. Those uses include:

- Anxiety
- Canker sores
- Fall prevention
- Hair loss
- Post-surgical pain

In "food amounts" lavender oil is rated "probably" safe. When used orally or applied directly to the skin, lavender oil earns a "possibly safe" rating.

Lavender oil should not be used on young boys or by pregnant or breast-feeding women. Any use of lavender should be stopped two weeks before any surgery.

The NIH urges caution for folks taking certain drugs, especially sedatives and medications for high blood pressure. That advice also applies to herbs and nutritional supplements. Supplements that could interact with lavender oil include:

- Cat's claw
- St. John's wort
- Stinging nettle
- Valerian

The agency makes no official dosage recommendation for lavender oil.

Monographs & Lavender Profiles:

Commission E. (1984). Lavender flower (Lavandulae flos). *Commission E Monographs*. English translation available online:
http://buecher.heilpflanzen-welt.de/BGA-Commission-E-Monographs/0224.htm

World Health Organization. (2009). Flos Lavandulae. *WHO Monographs On Selected Medicinal Plants, Volume 3*. Available online:
http://apps.who.int/medicinedocs/documents/s14213e/s14213e.pdf

European Medicines Agency. (2013). Lavender Oil. *Herbal Medicine: Summary For The Public*. Available online:
http://www.ema.europa.eu/ema/index.jsp?curl=pages/medicines/herbal/medicines/herbal_med_000121.jsp

National Institutes of Health. (2007). Lavender. *Herbs At A Glance*. Available online:
https://nccih.nih.gov/health/lavender/ataglance.htm

LAVENDER IN AROMATHERAPY

Ask five different aromatherapists to explain exactly how essential oils work to promote health and you might get five different answers. One person might tell you that essential oils work by stimulating the brain's limbic system, which, according to the theory, then spurs your body's natural healing ability.

The next person, though, might tell you that essential oils work more directly by killing harmful viruses, yeast or bacteria outright. He or she might cite one of the dozens of good scientific studies that have looked at essential oils and their effectiveness in the fight against harmful pathogens.

One of the newest explanations for how essential oils work "explains" that the oils "unclog" your cells' receptor sites, allowing your cells to better communicate with one another. Proponents of this theory sometimes claim that the process can also re-configure broken DNA.

A few aromatherapists even teach that essential oils are "alive", in a sense. This belief teaches that essential oils infuse you with the living energy of the plant from which they were made.

So if there is so little consensus on how volatile oils work, how can they agree on what lavender essential oil does in the body? That too, is debated but the uses for lavender essential oil can be grouped under three broad headings:

- Medical aromatherapy
- Holistic aromatherapy
- Emotional aromatherapy
- Perfumery

Medical Aromatherapy

Medical aromatherapy is the study of essential oils as replacements for, or adjuncts too, pharmaceutical drugs. There have been hundreds of scientific studies on lavender and its essential oil in mainstream medical journals.

In recent years studies on lavender essential oil have looked at it as a potential treatment for conditions like anxiety, insomnia, heart disease and postpartum mood issues.

Lavender oil has also shown promise in alleviating post-chemo nausea and as a way to reduce oxidative stress in diabetics. One study even suggested that lavender could help women suffering from heavy menstrual periods.

Holistic Aromatherapy

Practitioners of holistic aromatherapy also seek to replace at least some of our pharmaceuticals with volatile organic extracts but this practice is based on the belief that modern medicine, including its drugs, surgeries and focus on physical symptoms, are part of why we become ill in the first place.

In holistic aromatherapy lavender oil is perhaps most highly prized for its ability to affect the central nervous system but it is widely used for ailments affecting almost every part of the body.

According to today's aromatherapy authors, lavender has these beneficial actions on the body:

- Analgesic
- Antibacterial, antiviral and fungicidal
- Anticonvulsive
- Antispasmodic
- Antidepressant
- Carminative
- Cholagogue, diuretic and decongestant
- Deodorant and sudorific
- Emmenagogue
- Healing, antirheumatic, antiphlogistic, cell stimulative
- Hypotensive and sedative
- Restorative

Emotional Aromatherapy

All holistic aromatherapists believe that emotional wellbeing is just as vital to good health as physical wellbeing, but some go even further. Emotional aromatherapists believe that essential oils work even within the soul, "unclogging" the natural healing energy we each possess.

In emotional aromatherapy, lavender essential oil are thought to correspond to both feminine and masculine traits and is believed to act in whichever manner the user needs most. For example, for someone who is at the mercy of harmful or excessive stress, lavender will have a calming, sedative effect; for the person struggling with depression or emotional depletion, it will, aromatherapists say, have a stimulating, uplifting effect.

Some common uses for lavender oil in emotional aromatherapy include:

- Stress reduction
- Anxiety
- Insomnia caused by stress or anxiety
- Irritability

Perfumery

Millennia before the word "aromatherapy" entered our lexicon, humans were turning plants into perfumes and other scented products. For centuries, fragrant plants have helped us cleanse our sacred spaces, purify our minds and bury our dead. And while technology is allowing an increasing number of essential oils to be replaced with synthetic scents, plants remain perfumery's primary source materials.

In modern perfume production all lavenders are considered middle notes or middle-to-top notes. Middle notes like lavender make up the "heart" of a scent; they're sometimes referred to as the heart notes One of their primary purposes is to cover the initial odor of a perfume's "base" notes, allowing those notes, which can seem quite harsh in the first second or two that they're smelled, to develop a bit before they are perceived by the nose.

Traditionally, lavender has always been put into the fougère scent family.

In aromatherapy, lavender is one of the most "blendable" of all the essential oils. It blends especially well with citrus oils—bermagot, especially.

Popular Aromatherapy Books:

The Complete Guide to Aromatherapy by Salvatore Battaglia – This is the most "complete" guide of all the commonly available aromatherapy books in the US market. It is one of the few books on essential oils Lisa Barger ever personally recommended.

Aromatherapy for Healing the Spirit: Restoring Emotional and Mental Balance with Essential Oils by Gabriel Mojay – Mojay's book brought the concept of "emotional" aromatherapy into the mainstream market.

The Complete Book of Essential Oils and Aromatherapy by Valerie Worwood – This book is widely credited with helping to kick off the aromatherapy mania of the 1990s.

Advanced Aromatherapy: The Science of Essential Oil Therapy by Kurt Schnaubelt – When it was released, Schnaubelt's book was hailed as one of the first user-friendly aromatherapy guides to focus on the science of essential oils.

Gattefosse's Aromatherapy by Rene Maurice Gattefosse – This is Louise Davids' English-language translation of a book written by the man believed to have coined the word "aromatherapy" in the 1930s.

LAVENDER OIL MYTHS & SCAMS

The internet's offering of herbal medicine blog entries, social media posts and self-published booklets is rife with myths and scams that range from, at best, harmlessly untrue to, at worst, potentially dangerous. Whether it's written by well-meaning aromatherapy enthusiasts or scammers trying to sell you on a specific brand of aromatherapy products, most of this dubious information can be grouped into one of three categories:

- Info that is based on hearsay and folklore but which has no actual science behind it,
- Info that is based on scant science but which might be proven true, at least in part, as better information is discovered, and
- Outright lies and bent truths designed to entice you to buy essential oils—and buy them from a specific company.

Here are some of the common aromatherapy myths you'll find as you research essential oils on the 'net:

Lavender For Black Widow Spider Bites

One of the first aromatherapy books to get really popular here in the US, and the one that many credit with helping to rocket aromatherapy to super-fad status, referred to lavender oil as an antidote to black widow venom. To be fair, the author did say, "reportedly an antidote" but, judging from the myriad blog posts out there on using essential oils for spider bites and insect stings, it's clear that many people took her words as fact. It isn't at all difficult to find amateur herbalists recommending lavender for just such a purpose, even when the spider in question is a potentially deadly one.

The truth is that no scientific studies have ever even hinted at lavender oil's supposed ability to neutralize the latrotoxins in black widow venom. And, its primary chemical components—linalool, eucalyptol, linalyl acetate and camphor—also seem to offer no known anti-venom actions.

Lavender Oil And Cats

The book that calls lavender an antidote to spider venom also recommends using the oil on a variety of pets, including cats. The author is not alone in her thinking; some of the biggest names in aromatherapy have confessed to dropping a bit of lavender oil on their own cats from time to time.

But is lavender oil really safe for our feline friends? "No," says veterinarian Arnold Plotnick in a Q&A for the pet website CatChannel.com. Plotnick explains that after lavender oil is absorbed through your cat's skin it travels to your cat's liver, where the real trouble can begin. Cats cannot metabolize some very popular essential oils—including lavender—so the essential oil becomes a toxin in your cat's system. Lavender oil poisoning is such a concern that Plotnick even recommends avoiding petting a cat immediately after you've used certain toiletries—like a lavender-scented hand lotion.

You can read Dr. Plotnick's comments on lavender oil, in context, here: http://www.catchannel.com/media/experta/arnold_plotnick/plotnick-cat-lavender.aspx

Agreeing with Plotnick is veterinarian Jill Richardson. In 1999 she authored *Potpourri Hazards In Cats*, in which she shared a frightening bit of information about our pets and scented organic materials.

Between 1995 and 1999, she says, the ASPCA, or American Society for the Prevention of Cruelty to Animals, and its Animal Poison Control Center logged 125 reports of cats experiencing medical problems after they were exposed to liquid potpourri products, including botanicals that had been scented with natural extracts like essential oils.

You can read Dr. Richardson's piece here: http://aspcapro.org/sites/pro/files/zh-toxbrief_1299_0.pdf

Richardson's report didn't separate potpourris made with essential oils from those made with synthetic scents but a more recent report provided some pretty damning evidence against the use of lavender on cats.

That report, which also came from the ASPCA, documented thirty-nine cases of cats (and nine dogs) being sickened by "natural" flea remedies that injured the cats even when the person applying the flea treatment followed the product labels exactly.

In those cases, one cat died as a result of essential oil poisoning and another was ultimately euthanized. (One of the dogs was also euthanized.)

Lavender As A Germ Killer

The science is clear—lavender kills a wide variety of germs and dozens of studies prove it. But there's a big difference between saying, "Lavender kills germs," and claiming "You can disinfect your entire house with a few drops of lavender in your mop water."

A 2013 study in the *Iranian Journal of Medical Sciences* looked at various essential oils as a potential treatment for the bacterial disease brucellosis. Of the essential oils looked at in the study, lavender was not among those that showed promise against the *Brucella* bacterium.

That is typical of studies that compare lavender oils against oils like clove, thyme and cinnamon, which have long been considered potent germ killers. In study after study, lavender has proven itself useful against some of our most dangerous pathogens but it isn't effective against all germs and it isn't always the best choice for any particular bacterium, virus or fungus.

"Therapy Grade"/"Aromatherapy Grade" Lavender Essential Oil

Despite what some aromatherapy sellers will tell you, there is no official grading system for essential oils, either here in the US or in Europe. And don't be fooled by registered trademarks, either, which you can identify with this symbol: ®. It's just a company's way of trying to convince you that its line of essential oils is the best.

That doesn't mean that companies who use "therapeutic grade" claims, or even registered trademarks are trying to trick you. There *are* brands that source their essential oils with specific chemical goals in mind. To them, "therapeutic grade" might mean that the plants are grown under very specific conditions or that the distillation process is done at a specific temperature.

The important thing to remember is that, legally, claims like "aromatherapy grade" and "therapy grade" are meaningless.

"You can't be allergic to lavender (or any other) essential oil."

One of the most hurtful scams in aromatherapy—because it ultimately blames YOU for your discomfort instead of the product—is the one that says pure essential oils are not capable of causing reactions like rashes, breakouts or headaches. The exact explanations vary but, generally, they include reasoning like:

- If you have an allergic reaction to lavender oil it means your oil isn't pure. It's probably been adulterated.
- If you get a headache from smelling lavender it means the oil is detoxing you. It is your body's own stored toxins that are making you sick.
- Lavender oil is simply not capable of triggering an allergy because allergies are triggered by proteins and essential oils don't contain proteins.

The most common argument is likely the one about purity. You see this most often being claimed by sales representatives of multi-level-marketing, or MLM, companies. Essential oils can certainly vary in quality but, ultimately, this argument is nothing more than an attempt to convince you that a particular company's lavender oil is somehow superior in quality to another company's.

The truth is, scientists now believe they know which of the compounds in lavender oil cause topical reactions like contact dermatitis but those substances are not impurities. They are naturally occurring compounds—and they just happen to be the ones believed to be lavender essential oil's "active" components.

The "toxins" explanation is a retelling of a myth long-used by herbalists. "If an herb makes you feel nauseated, gives you a headache, or causes your skin to break out, that's a good sign. It means it's forcing toxins out of your body." Yet aromatherapists who spread this myth never quite seem to get around to explaining exactly what those toxins are or what, exactly, the lavender oil is doing in the body to cause such a sudden and dramatic purge. There is no science to support such claims.

So what about the claim that allergic reactions require proteins? Think about all the metals that are known to cause allergic responses. Nickel is perhaps the most widely known but gold and chromium are two more examples of common metals capable of causing allergic reactions—and none of them contain protein.

Reference:

Worwood, V. (1991). *The Complete Book of Essential Oils & Aromatherapy.* New World Library.

Plotnick, A. (No date given). *Are Lavender Scented Products Harmful to My Cat?* Available online:
http://www.catchannel.com/experts/arnold_plotnick/plotnick-cat-lavender.aspx

Richardson, J. (1999). Potpourri Hazards in Cats. *Veterinary Medicine.* Available online:
http://www.aspcapro.org/sites/pro/files/zh-toxbrief_1299_0.pdf

Genovese, A., et al. (2012). Adverse Reactions from Essential Oil-Containing Natural Flea Products Exempted From Environmental Protection Agency Regulations in Dogs and Cats. *Journal of Veterinary Emergency and Critical Care.* Abstract available online:
http://www.ncbi.nlm.nih.gov/pubmed/22805458

Al-Mariri, A., et al. (2013). The Antibacterial Activity of Selected Labiatae (Lamiaceae) Essential Oils against Brucella melitensis. *Iranian Journal of Medical Sciences.* Available online:
http://europepmc.org/articles/PMC3642944

Streicher, C. (No date given). *Amrita's Purity Standards.* Available online:
https://www.amrita.net/amrita-aromatherapy-purity-standards

FINDING GOOD LAVENDER ESSENTIAL OIL

Lavender is a lovely choice for someone looking to incorporate "natural" scents into the home. Sorting through the myriad brands that are out there, though, can be overwhelming, especially if volatile oils are new to you.

Finding Quality Essential Oils

How do you know you're getting what you think you're paying for when you buy one of those little bottles of lavender essential oil at your supermarket, pharmacy or health food store? How can you be sure that the lavender you're buying is really lavender and completely pure?

The blunt truth is, you can't. But you can stack the odds in your favor by looking at how ethical aromatherapy companies produce, package and label their products:

- Botanical nomenclature – "Lavender" can mean any species in the *Lavandula* genus. An ethical producer will tell you exactly which species you're buying—and do it in the generally accepted way of listing both the genus and species, with the genus capitalized and the species in lowercase.
- Essential oil declaration – Essential oils such say something like, "Essential Oil" or "100% Pure Essential" on their labels. If they do not, or they say something like "perfume" or "scent", they may not be pure volatile oils.
- Specialization – Terms like "certified" and "therapy grade" are really just marketing spiel. Look past the legally toothless claims and choose brands produced specifically for aromatherapy. That usually

means that those products are distilled at lower temperatures—a factor considered especially important for essential oils like lavender.

- Opaque bottles – Volatile oil producers agree that opaque bottles are must-haves to stop sunlight from accelerating the natural oxidation process.

A company doesn't list its parent plant, its country of origin or make a big deal about being produced specifically for aromatherapy use isn't necessarily trying to cheat you. But a company that *does* do those things is saying to you that it recognizes your commitment to quality and that it's willing to be a bit more accountable than some of its competitors.

Debunking The "Clean Evaporation" Test

A number of aromatherapy authors recommend a simple to test to determine whether your essential oil is pure. It goes like this: Drop a single drop of your essential oil onto a piece of plain white paper and wait for it to dry. If the essential oil evaporates without leaving behind a residue or a stain, it will prove that your essential oil is pure.

While it's true that most distilled essential oils will evaporate without staining a piece of white paper, the "clean evaporation" test is not a reliable test of purity for any essential oil.

First, it ignores that fact that in most cases—and this is especially true with lavender essential oil—the most common adulterants are not synthetic chemicals that will leave behind some kind of residue. The most common adulterants are other essential oils.

In fact, most common way to adulterate lavender oil is actually to blend a high-quality lavender—like *L. angustifolia*, for example, with an essential oil distilled from a cheaper, faster growing species of lavender. In those cases, the evaporation test will be completely useless.

Second, the "clean evaporation" test ignores the fact that a few essential oils simply are not clear, no matter how "pure" they are. There is a species of chamomile, for example, that yields a brilliant blue volatile oil.

To some degree, an essential oil buyer is at the mercy of the supplier. An ethical supplier will do what it can to earn your trust and won't rely on sales spiel and gimmicks.

LAVENDER ESSENTIAL OIL IN YOUR HOME

When it comes to how you scent your home with volatile oils, the choices can seem overwhelming, especially if you are new to aromatherapy.

But it doesn't have be. All aromatherapy diffusers—from those little cloth light bulb rings to the big plug-in diffusers that are attached to air pumps—fall into one of two categories:

- Passive diffusers
- Active diffusers

Passive diffusers work by allowing essential oils to evaporate naturally. Dropping a few drops of lavender essential oil into a bowl of potpourri is the classic example of using passively diffused scent. Using heat—buy dropping your lavender essential oil into one of those little miniature crock-style cookers, for example—is an example of using active diffusing scent.

The method—or methods—you choose to scent your space will depend on how much money you're willing to invest, how "hands on" you want to get and how safety-minded you need to be.

Passive Aromatherapy Diffusers

Passive aromatherapy diffusers are popular because they tend to low-tech, easy to use and relatively inexpensive.
- An old bowl of potpourri makes a wonderful and inexpensive passive diffuser. Just drop a few drops of lavender essential oil onto the dried plant material and place the bowl out of reach of pets and

children.

- A cotton ball stuffed into an old shot glass is easily tucked into a curio cabinet or bookshelf. Drop a few drops of lavender onto the cotton ball and tuck your homemade diffuser out of sight.
- Combat garbage can odors by soaking a piece of tissue or paper towel with lavender and dropping into your trash can.

Active Aromatherapy Diffusers

Active aromatherapy diffusers accelerate the dispersal of essential oil vapors through mechanical means—and often, though not always, with heat.

- Metal lamp rings with lavender added to their reservoirs sit atop your light bulbs and disperse scent as heat from the bulb is given off.
- Miniature crock-style diffusers filled with water to which a few drops of lavender essential oil is added both scents and gently humidifies your space.
- Specially made aroma balls plug right into a wall outlet; they use tiny fiber pads to hold essential oil droplets over a small warming plate.
- Candle diffusers both light and scent your space by using a tea light candle to warm a small, essential-oil-filled bowl suspended above it.

Also in the "active" category are the nebulizing diffusers. These electrically powered diffusers typically use no heat; they force air into a reservoir, forcing out a vaporized mist of scent.

So which diffuser is right for you? That will depend upon how much money you want to spend, how much time you're willing to spend and the unique safety considerations your home requires.

Candle diffusers, for example, create instant ambiance in the evenings but you wouldn't want to place one where children or pets could get to it. Crock-style warmers can run for hours, adding a bit of humidity to the air as they do, but again, there's that scald risk.

Nebulizing diffusers make very efficient use of your essential oils but they're quite expensive, require special and careful cleaning and, because they are powered by an electric motor, are loud.

Whichever diffusion method you choose, there will be maintenance and safety considerations. You know your family and your home best. Choose the diffuser that fits into your lifestyle.

Diffusing Lavender Safely In Your Home

It is important to remember the old saying, "It might be natural but that doesn't mean it's harmless." Just as even the purist lavender essential oil can harm you, a single stray drop can ruin finished wood, warp plastic appliances and mar and destroy other surfaces in your home.

And it isn't just your tabletops and hardwood floors that should fear lavender, either. The inside of your dishwasher, the dispenser cups in your washer and dryer, the bladder in your carpet shampooer . . . even the plastic parts of your vacuum cleaner can be damaged by essential oils.

Of course, there is also the issue of accidental poisonings from essential oils. While exact numbers are hard to come by, there have been documented cases of pets being poisoned after consuming potpourri and children being sickened after consuming essential oils. (Most essential oils are not packaged in child resistant containers.)

LAVENDER TOXICITY & SAFETY ISSUES

Lavender essential oil is aromatherapy's darling when it comes to the issue of safety. It is not, however, completely non-toxic or non-irritating, as some devoted lavender lovers claim. There are many documented cases of people being injured or sickened by the herb and its oil:

Skin Reactions

Not everyone shares aromatherapy's opinion of lavender as a completely safe essential oil. A 2004 study in *Cell Proliferation* claimed that *in vitro* tests on lavender dilutions as low as 0.25% were cytotoxic to human skin cells. The researchers theorized that the oil damages skin by first weakening your cells' membranes.

A 20015 study in the journal *Contact Dermatitis* looked at numerous herbs employed as "natural" remedies in Europe and their history of causing contact dermatitis. It found that even at 16% concentration, lavender oil was safe for direct skin contact, although it noted 2 cases of dermatitis that were ultimately linked to pillows made with dried lavender flowers. Both of the patients had used pure essential oil to "refresh" the pillows' scents.

The study's authors then speculated that the real culprit in allergic-type skin reactions is oxidation of three chemical components:

- Linalool
- Linalyl acetate
- Geraniol

Those types of reactions will only become more frequent, say the authors of a 2011 study in the journal *Dermatitis*. In Japan, cases of contact dermatitis linked to lavender essential oil exposure increased thirteen-fold in 8 years as aromatherapy and aromatherapy massages became popular.

Gynecomastia

When doctors, writing in a 2007 issue of *New England Journal of Medicine,* linked lavender-scented toiletries to gynecomastia, or abnormal breast development, in three young brothers the news frightened a lot of people—including many people in the aromatherapy industry.

Many in the aromatherapy world refused to believe that the amount of lavender oil absorbed from bath soap and hand lotion could possibly act as so potent an endocrine disruptor that it could cause symptoms like the one doctors described. Some even claimed that lavender oil wasn't capable of doing that at all. Maybe it wasn't the lavender but the plastic packaging, one group claimed. Perhaps it was something the boys ate, like too much licorice or maybe too many garbanzo beans, suggested the founder of an essential oil company.

The authors stood by their original findings, though, and in 2010 published more research, this time in the journal *Hormones.* That study found that lavender oil certainly *could* act as a hormone disruptor and that the effect was dose dependent. It also underlined the need for more research on the potential dangers similar products could pose as consumers' preferences for "natural" cosmetics and toiletries continues to grow.

Tachycardia

In 2011 doctors in Turkey treated a middle-aged woman for low blood pressure, rapid heartbeat and shortness of breath. Several hours before making her way to the emergency room, she told them, she had consumed a tea made from lavender herb. Her symptoms began, she said, about an hour later and, at the time of her admission to the emergency room, had been going on for about six hours.

The authors of this study believe that it was the camphor in the tea that caused the patient's symptoms. The species of lavender, *L. stoechas*, is typically high in camphor.

This is believed to be the first time tachycardia, or a high resting heart rate, has been blamed on lavender products.

Reference:

Prashar, A., et al. (2004). Cytotoxicity of Lavender Oil and its Major Components to Human Skin Cells. *Cell Proliferation*. Abstract available: http://www.ncbi.nlm.nih.gov/pubmed/15144499

Gangemi, S., et al. (2015). Contact Dermatitis as an Adverse Reaction to some Topically Ssed European Herbal Medicinal Products - part 2: Echinacea purpurea-Lavandula angustifolia. *Contact Dermatitis*. Available online:
http://onlinelibrary.wiley.com/doi/10.1111/cod.12328/epdf

Wu, P., e al. (2011). Lavender. *Dermatitis*. Abstract available:
http://www.ncbi.nlm.nih.gov/pubmed/22653008

Henley, D., et al. (2007). Prepubertal Gynecomastia Linked to Lavender and Tea Tree Oils. *New England Journal of Medicine*. Available online:
http://www.nejm.org/doi/full/10.1056/nejmoa064725

Henley, D., et al. (2010). Physiological Effects and Mechanisms of Action of Endocrine Disrupting Chemicals that Alter Estrogen Signaling. *Hormones*. Available online:
http://www.hormones.gr/pdf/HORMONES%202010%20191-205.pdf

Acikalin, A., et al. (2011). Anticholinergic Syndrome and Supraventricular Tachycardia Caused by Lavender Tea Toxicity. *The Keio Journal of Medicine*. Available online:
https://www.jstage.jst.go.jp/article/kjm/61/2/61_66/_pdf

SCIENTIFIC STUDIES ON LAVENDER OIL

You've heard the myth: "Doctor's don't prescribe herbs because they don't know anything about them. That's because no one studies herbs; there's no money in natural remedies."

The truth is, "natural" medicines like herbs, and essential oils made from herbs, are being studied every day. The results of the good studies—the double-blind, peer-reviewed studies--are being published in major medical journals. The science on essential oils isn't being suppressed by some government agency. Nor is it relegated to obscure, niche journals.

In fact, in just the past five years, lavender and its essential oil have been studied as potential treatments for such diverse medical issues as:

- Insomnia
- Anxiety
- "Superbug" infections
- Stroke
- Diabetes
- Dementia

Lavender For Better Sleep

A 2015 study done at University of Minnesota's School of Nursing looked at lavender oil and whether its scent could improve sleep quality for college students who had previously reported having trouble sleeping.

What the researchers did was to put chest patches on 96 volunteers and tracked, for 5 days, how well the students slept while using wearable fitness trackers and keeping sleep diaries. Half of the volunteers got patches infused with lavender essential oil while the rest of them wore "blanks". All the volunteers were encouraged to practice good sleep hygiene.

At the end of the study the scientists discovered that the volunteers who had worn the lavender patches experienced better quality sleep than those who wore the blanks. The lavender benefit even lasted through the two week follow-up period.

It isn't just college students who may benefit from the sleep enhancing effects of lavender. An Iranian study found that new mothers may also rest better with a bit of lavender in their space.

This study involved 158 postpartum women, half of whom were given containers of lavender-scented balls to smell immediately before lying down to sleep. The women were instructed to inhale the lavender aroma, taking 10 deep breaths, 4 times a week for 8 weeks. At the time, the women's sleep quality was scored and found to have been improved enough in the lavender users to leave the researchers with the conclusion that lavender essential oil, smelled at bedtime, could be "effective at improving sleeping in new mothers and a drug-free way to improve their overall wellbeing."

Lavender For Anxiety

Of all the health concerns lavender is supposed to treat, it is, perhaps, anxiety for which science offers the most documentation. One of the most recent studies on lavender for anxiety was published in 2014 and focused on the exact biological mechanisms that go into making lavender oil so effective. What the researchers discovered was that lavender works by, in their words, "significantly increasing" levels of the neurotransmitter serotonin in the brain. Serotonin does several things in the body, including increasing feelings of well-being.

This study also supported previous research that has suggested it isn't just the smell of lavender that makes people feel better. Some of the mice in this study had their sense of smell destroyed before they were exposed to the oil; they experienced increased serotonin levels, despite not being able to perceive the lavender aroma at all.

Lavender For Dementia

Lavender has long been used as a sleep aid and as an anti-anxiety remedy so in 2013 researchers recruited 12 nurses to test whether lavender could be an effective treatment for people suffering from sleep problems and anxiety cause by dementia. After diffusing oil made from "true" lavender, or *Lavandula angustifolia*, into the air, nurses at all 4 of the nursing homes reported the patients slept better and were less anxious.

The only problems noted in this very small study were experienced by the nurses themselves, who found themselves having to explain the basics of aromatherapy to skeptical coworkers.

Lavender For Wounds, Burns And Skin Health

The man who gave us the word "aromatherapy" is also the man who popularized lavender as a wound healer. René-Maurice Gattefossé claims to have discovered lavender oil's power after he used it to treat a badly infected hand, which had become gangrenous after being burned in a lab accident.

Afraid of losing his hand, Gattefossé "instinctively", as he put it, treated his wound with lavender. The gangrene was cured, the burns healed, and Gattefossé went on to become known as the father of modern aromatherapy.

For decades the Gattefossé story has been repeated, and embellished, until it's impossible to know exactly how important the lavender really was. But even if the story is little more than a charming legend, there's likely some truth in it. In 2014 a group of researchers in the Slovak Republic actually tested 15 different essential oils against several *Clostridium* bacteria—the very bacteria responsible for most cases of gas gangrene.

 Of the oils tested, the oil made from *Lavandula angustifolia* came in at just over 90% inhibition after 30 minutes. That was good enough to best all other oils in the study, except oils of oregano and winter savory.

This was not the first study to look at lavender as a treatment for life-threatening infections. A recent study from Morocco looked at the essential oil of *Lavandula coronopifolia*, or stag's horn lavender, as a way to fight several types of bacteria that are quickly becoming resistant to standard pharmaceutical antibiotics. At dilutions as weak as 1% the stag's horn lavender oil showed at least some ability to fight these "superbugs".

Lavender For Diabetes

The exact role the toxin alloxan plays in the development of diabetes in humans—if it even plays a role at all—is controversial but that didn't stop

Tunisian researchers from looking at *Lavandula stoechas* as a potential diabetes treatment in 2013. They made laboratory rats diabetic with alloxan, which destroyed the rats' insulin cells and then treated the animals with the essential oil, which they distilled themselves, for 15 days. The lavender-treated rats achieved better glucose control and experienced less oxidative stress. The scientists behind this study credit the results to the antioxidant activity of the lavender oil.

In 2015 that same team of researchers repeated their experiments, this time including rosemary essential oil—also with positive results.

Lavender For Stroke

A handful of studies have looked recently at lavender oil for stroke victims. One was published in 2012 and found that it could protect stroke victims' brains from the loss of blood and the injuries caused when blood returns to the damaged part of the brain. The mice in this study had better post-stroke cognitive scores, smaller damage sites and healthier brain chemistry if they were treated with lavender oil.

More recently, scientists looked at lavender oil specifically as a potential treatment for swelling in the brain. Again, this was an animal study but the results suggest that lavender might reduce the size of the area destroyed and improve neurological functions. Lavender did not, however, actually stop the process of apoptosis, or cell death in the brain.

Reference:

Lillehei, A., et al. (2015). Effect of Inhaled Lavender and Sleep Hygiene on Self-Reported Sleep Issues: A Randomized Controlled Trial. *The Journal of Alternative and Complementary Medicine*. Abstract available online:
http://online.liebertpub.com/doi/10.1089/acm.2014.0327

Keshavarz, A., et al. (2015). Lavender fragrance essential oil and the quality of sleep in postpartum women. *Iranian Red Crescent Medical Journal*. Available online:
http://www.ncbi.nlm.nih.gov/pmc/articles/PMC4443384/

Takahashi, M., et al. (2014). Anxiolytic-like Effect of Inhalation of Essential Oil from Lavandula officinalis: Investigation of Changes in 5-HT Turnover and Involvement of Olfactory Stimulation. *Natural Product Communications*. Abstract available online:
http://www.ncbi.nlm.nih.gov/pubmed/25230519

Johannessen, B. (2013). Nurses Experience of Aromatherapy use with Dementia Patients Experiencing Disturbed Sleep Patterns. An Action Research Project. *Complementary Therapies In Clinical Practice*. Abstract available online:
http://www.ncbi.nlm.nih.gov/pubmed/24199975

Kačániová, M., et al. (2014). Antibacterial Activity against Clostridium genus and Antiradical Activity of the Essential Oils from Different Origin. *Journal of Environmental Science and Health*. Abstract available online:
http://www.ncbi.nlm.nih.gov/pubmed/24813985

Said, A., et al. (2015). Chemical Composition and Antibacterial Activity of Lavandula coronopifolia Essential Oil against Antibiotic-Resistant Bacteria. *Natural Product Research*. Abstract available online:
http://www.ncbi.nlm.nih.gov/pubmed/25174508

Sebai, H., et al. (2013). Lavender (Lavandula stoechas L.) Essential Oils Attenuate Hyperglycemia and Protect against Oxidative Stress in Alloxan-Induced Diabetic Rats. *Lipids in Health and Disease*. Available online:
http://lipidworld.biomedcentral.com/articles/10.1186/1476-511X-12-189

Sebai, H., et al. (2015). Protective Effect of Lavandula stoechas and Rosmarinus officinalis Essential Oils Against Reproductive Damage and Oxidative Stress in Alloxan-Induced Diabetic Rats. *Journal of Medicinal Food*. Abstract available online:
http://online.liebertpub.com/doi/abs/10.1089/jmf.2014.0040

Wang, D., et al. (2012). Neuroprotective Activity of Lavender Oil on Transient Focal Cerebral Ischemia in Mice. *Molecules*. Abstract available online:
http://www.mdpi.com/1420-3049/17/8/9803

Vakili, A., (2014). Effect of Lavender Oil (Lavandula angustifolia) on Cerebral Edema and its Possible Mechanisms in an Experimental Model of Stroke. *Brain Research*. Abstract available:
http://www.ncbi.nlm.nih.gov/pubmed/24384140

LAVENDER WATERS & HYDROSOLS

Sold alongside essential oils are other scented products, including floral waters and hydrosols.

Lavender Waters

Floral waters, which are correctly referred to as herbal distillates, are the co-products of the distillation process. Lavender water is the condensate left in the still's collection chamber after the essential oil has been skimmed off.

Lavender water is often bulk-packaged and sold to cosmetics and toiletries manufacturers to be used in the production of soap, lotions and other skin care products. It is also sold for use as a facial toner, an air freshener or bed linen spray.

Lavender Hydrosols

Aromatherapist Jeanne Rose claims to have coined the term "hydrosol" after imagining lavender plants growing between grapevines in a vineyard. She opines that a quality hydrosol, which uses only the first 25% or so of the condensate, is "20-30 times more concentrated" than an herbal tea.

Hydrosols can be used as-is on the skin or packaged for use in cosmetics and toiletries. Rose also recommend the consumption of certain hydrosols.

So What's The Difference?

All hydrosols are floral waters but, at least according to Jeanne Rose and her followers, not all floral waters are high enough quality to be called "hydrosol".

LAVANDINS & LAVENDER BLENDS

Occasionally you'll see something labeled "Lavandin Oil" or a label that refers to its contents as a "Blend of Lavender".

Lavandin Essential Oils

Lavandins are not fancy new species of lavender; they are simply hybrids. Most often they are hybrids of *Lavandula angustifolia* and either *L. lanata* or *L. latifolia*.

Lavandin essential oils tend to be a bit cheaper than "true" lavender essential oils and can smell a bit harsher to the nose.

Lavender Essential Oil Blends

Some essential oil producers prefer to blend their lavenders. Blending can an aromatic choice, as in the case of a producer who simply wishes to "harden" a particularly "sweet" batch or it can be a way to save money by "cutting" an expensive batch with a variety that is a bit more cost effective.

Using blends also allows growers to adopt a use-what-you-have approach to each individual growing season. As with any crop, lavender yields vary from season to season. Blends can be a handy way for small growers, especially, to maximize those yields.

Like lavandin essential oils, lavender blends tend to be less expensive for the consumer.

"THANK YOU!" FOR READING

Thank you for reading *Lavender Essential Oil*. If you enjoyed this booklet, please consider leaving a review on the website of your favorite book seller. Your feedback helps us understand what you liked, what you didn't like—and what we should improve. Other readers will thank you, too.

ABOUT THE AUTHOR

Lisa Barger has been called "one of our greatest educators in the alternative medicine field" and someone who is "on a mission" to debunk myths and expose charlatans with a "pit bull energy".

She is the founder and principal writer at the LisaBarger.com family of websites, covering food safety, natural health scams, infant product recalls and more.

Her columns are syndicated through Amazon's Kindle Blogs.

Lisa currently lives in Cabot, Arkansas.

www.ingramcontent.com/pod-product-compliance
Lightning Source LLC
Chambersburg PA
CBHW030546290526
45786CB00004B/1893